The Layman's Guide to Medical School

Inside the Human Cell

Text copyright © 2015 Colleen Fleshman.
All rights reserved.
§
This book is not intended as a substitute for the medical advice of physicians. The reader should regularly consult a physician in matters relating to his/her health and particularly with respect to any symptoms that may require diagnosis or medical attention.

INTRODUCTION	4
THE BODY	5
THE STRUCTURE OF THE CELL	10
DNA	17
CELL REPLICATION	24
THE NUCLEUS	39
ORGANELLES	44
CELL SIGNALING	57
CELL DEATH	60
CONCLUSION	63
SOURCES	64

INTRODUCTION

The human body is composed of about 37 trillion cells, a number so large it's nearly impossible to comprehend. Luckily for us, the largest cell in the body—the female egg—is only about 120 μm in diameter, just about the smallest size the human eye can possibly see. Most cells in the body are much smaller, so they're invisible to the naked eye. Despite their miniscule size, though, the cells in our body are responsible for keeping us alive at every second of every day—a task I, frankly, don't envy.

So how do our cells function, and how do they keep us alive? That topic is what we'll explore in this book. *Inside the Human Cell* is intended as an introduction to the human cell, not a comprehensive review. Thousands of pages can be, and have been, written about the function of the cell. This book is intended to give you an understanding of the cell and its basic functions that can serve as a guide for future study on how the human body works. If you're interested in reading more, *Molecular Biology of the Human Cell* is an excellent textbook that I used in my undergrad Cell Biology course, though it'll take you a lot longer to read than this book. I hope you all enjoy the book, and if you have any questions, you can contact me at laymansmedicalschool@gmail.com.

THE BODY

In order to understand how cells work, it's important to understand the context in which cells live. Human cells don't live and function independently; they are all part of a very complex network of cells within the body that communicate with one another. Because cells are part of a team, they're able to specialize into different tissue types with specific roles. While the roles differ, the way in which the cell actually functions is more or less the same across all types of cells. This will make more sense as we get further in our understanding of the cell. One way to think about this is to think about people. We all eat, sleep, drink, and move the same basic way, but we're going in seven billion different directions at any given time. The cells function in the same way. They get energy and interact with the world around them in similar ways, but they're each performing different functions.

The question, of course, is, what are those functions? The types of cells in the body are very loosely divided into four types of tissues. "Tissue" refers to a group of cells and their products that perform a similar function. These four types are nervous, muscular, epithelial, and connective. We'll look at each one of these in more detail.

Nervous tissue refers to the cells that make up the nervous system, a network of cells that send signals through your body so quickly that you aren't aware of any delay between thought and movement. The nervous system, which is composed of the central nervous system—the brain and spinal cord—and the peripheral nervous system—all of the other nerves in the body that send messages to the periphery. There are two types of cells in the nervous system: the neurons and glial cells. Neurons are the communicating cells of the nervous system. These cells signal to one another, using mechanisms we won't get into right now, in order to pass messages along from one part of your body to the next. For instance, as you read this book, light reflecting off the page is activating a neuron in the back of your eye, which sends a long projection (called an axon) through the optic nerve that runs out the back of your eye to your brain. In the brain, this axon synapses with more neurons that form the visual cortex, which in turn send axons to another part of your brain that processes the information and translates the light signals into words. Meanwhile, another part of your brain is sending axons out to the muscles around your eye, called extra-ocular muscles, in order to move your eyes along the page. Yet another part sends axons to your heart and diaphragm, telling your heart to keep beating and your diaphragm to keep contracting so you breathe. Because these neurons have developed to send signals rapidly, you aren't even aware that this is happening. You simply think to take a step or stretch out an arm, and you do.

      The other type of cell found in nervous tissue is called a glial cell. Glial cells are the supporting cells of the nervous system. They don't send signals themselves, but they provide support for the neurons by providing protection (such as in the blood-brain barrier, which is partly composed of a type of glial cell called astrocytes that prevent most molecules from crossing out of the blood into the brain) and creating sheaths over the axons to speed up the signals that travel via these axons, among other things. The glial cells have a less glamorous job but are critical to the function of our nervous system. This becomes apparent in diseases such as multiple sclerosis, which destroys the glial cells, called oligodendrocytes, that create sheaths in the central nervous system.

The second type of tissue is probably one that you're familiar with, and this is muscular tissue. Muscular tissue, as you may have guessed, is what comprises every muscle in our body, from the large leg muscles that make up our quads to the tiny muscles that help with the fine movement of our fingers. Muscular tissue is specialized to contract, which is how muscles move. Think about flexing your arm at the elbow. You think to move your hand up, and the nerves send a signal down to the biceps muscle in your upper arm, which contracts. When the muscle contracts, it shortens, pulling on the bone it's attached to. At the same time, your brain sends a signal to your triceps muscle, inhibiting its contraction. This relaxes any pull to keep your arm straightened, and your forearm moves up.

There are three types of muscular tissue: skeletal muscle, smooth muscle, and cardiac muscle. Skeletal muscle, or striated muscle, makes up the muscles in your body that are under voluntary control, meaning you can move them at will. This includes all of the muscles in your arms and legs, as well as a number of muscles in your trunk, neck, and face. The "striated" part of this muscle name comes from the fact that the cells line up in a row with various densities of protein filaments, and the change in density and type of filament gives the muscle a striped (striated) appearance. Cardiac muscle is also a type of striated muscle, though it's not under voluntary control. As you can probably guess, cardiac muscle is found only in the heart and has special connections between the cells, called gap junctions, which allow signals to travel almost instantaneously through the cells so they all contract at the same time, leading to the outflow of blood from your heart. The final type of muscle tissue is smooth muscle, which makes up all muscle not under voluntary control, such as the muscle in your gastrointestinal tract that moves food along its path.

Epithelial tissue is less well known by name but is vastly important to the everyday function of your body. Epithelial tissue covers nearly all body surfaces and serves to protect the underlying tissue. The skin that covers our body is a type of epithelial tissue. These cells can also form glands that secrete substances, such as the glands in your airways that secrete mucus to protect them from harmful chemicals in the air. The last role of epithelial tissue is to absorb substances. This is most commonly seen in the gastrointestinal tract, where specialized epithelial cells called enterocytes absorb small sugar, protein, and fat molecules and release them into the blood to get transported to the rest of your body.

The final type of tissue is connective, which serves to keep the form of organs in your body. Any cells that support or connect tissue fall under this category. This includes the collagen you can feel in your nose and ears; collagen also provides a structure for bone to grow.

Ligaments and tendons are composed of connective tissue. The matrix that holds all cells together, aptly named the extracellular matrix, is connective tissue. One last important type of connective tissue is blood, which serves to bring nutrients, oxygen, and your immune cells to all of the tissues in your body.

Knowing the types of cells can help us understand how the body works as a whole, but to really understand how cells work, we need to zoom in on the cell itself.

THE STRUCTURE OF THE CELL

Now that we understand a bit about the tissues in the body, it's time to zoom in on the tiny functional units that comprise each tissue: the cell. Keep in mind that we're only talking about the human cell here, though most other animals have similar cell structure and function.

Each cell is made up of three main parts: the plasma membrane, the cytoplasm, and the nucleus. The plasma membrane is a—you guessed it—membrane that encloses the cell, protecting it from the outside environment. Inside the cell, there's another, smaller membrane enclosing a smaller area, known as the nucleus. The nucleus contains the DNA of the cell, which is the blueprint for making everything in the body. We'll talk more about the DNA in a later chapter. And finally, the cytoplasm is the fluid that fills the space between the nucleus and the plasma membrane.

The plasma membrane serves a far more important role than just enclosing the cell. This membrane decides how and when the cell communicates with the rest of the body, which we'll delve into in the section on cell signaling. For now, it's important to understand the composition of the membrane.

The majority of the membrane is made up of something

commonly called the lipid bilayer. Lipids are a group of substances that include fat, cholesterol, wax, and steroids, as well as a number of other substances that are related by the fact that they're insoluble in water. If you're familiar with chemistry, you'll know that substances can generally be grouped into two categories: hydrophobic and hydrophilic. Hydrophobic substances, like fat, don't dissolve in water. If you've ever poured oil and water together, you'll know what this looks like. On the other hand, hydrophilic substances, like sugar, dissolve when mixed with water. Without getting into too much chemistry, just know that this has to do with the fact that some elements have a stronger affinity for the electrons that are shared between the elements in a molecule than others. In the case of water, oxygen has a much stronger pull on the electrons than hydrogen does, so the electrons, which are negatively charged, sit closer to oxygen than to hydrogen. Molecules such as these are known as polar molecules. Since water is polar, other molecules that are also polar prefer to be surrounded by water. On the other hand, molecules that are composed of elements with similar affinities for the electrons are nonpolar. This is the case with fats, which are primarily composed of carbons. As you can imagine, carbons all have the same affinity for electrons since they're all the same. This makes the fats nonpolar, and therefore hydrophobic.

While lipids often get a bad reputation because of their role in heart disease, they're also vital to our survival (just not in the large doses we like to eat).

The majority of the cell membrane is made up of a specific type of lipid called phospholipids. These molecules are unique in that they have both a hydrophobic end and a hydrophilic end. This is possible because phospholipids are long molecules, usually made up of a chain of sixteen or more carbons. In comparison, water is only three atoms (the most basic unit that something can be broken down into and still retain the properties of the whole)—two hydrogens and an oxygen. Therefore, when a few charged atoms are added to one end of the chain, that end becomes hydrophilic and likes to bond with water via its polar charges. This is known as the head of the phospholipid, and is the part that contains the phosphate. The chain, also known as the tail, is nonpolar and therefore wants nothing to do with water. This property turns out to be vastly important in creating cells because the phospholipids tend to group together, with the tails (there are actually two per phospholipid) hanging out with the other tails to get away from the water, and the heads pointing outward to be closer to the water. When a second layer is added on the inside, the tails are protected on every side from the water, while the heads are exposed to the water. The structure looks something like this:

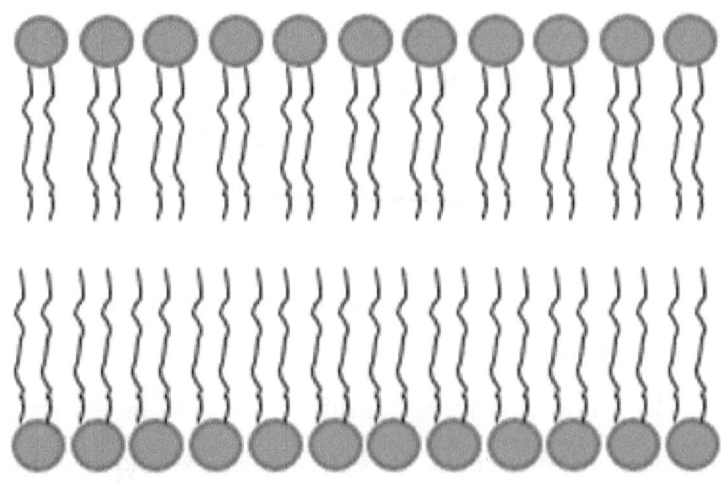

You can probably imagine now how the membrane curves around, forming a complete sphere so the tails are all inside the protection provided by the polar heads. The amphipathic nature of phospholipids allows cell membranes to form. One of the advantages to this structure is that it is fairly fluid, meaning that the cell's shape can change without destroying the integrity of the cell. You can imagine the cell membrane as a poorly filled balloon. When you press on the balloon, it indents without popping. Our cells can do the same thing when outside forces act on them.

While the majority of molecules in the membrane are phospholipids, there are other molecules in there. One such molecule is cholesterol, which helps the phospholipids pack more tightly together and therefore makes the membrane less fluid. This is useful to a certain degree, but too much cholesterol in the cell membrane can make it brittle and easily damaged, which kills the cell. The other, critical component of the cell membrane is proteins.

Proteins are the result of DNA transcription to RNA, which is then translated to proteins (more on this in the next chapter). Proteins can take on a wide variety of roles in the body, including acting as enzymes for reactions, breaking down food into nutrients we can absorb, absorbing those molecules, and on and on. In the case of cell membranes, proteins are so important that we've dedicated an entire chapter to their role in interacting with the world outside the cell. For now, we'll just say that proteins can be attached to the cell membrane in one of two ways: either as a peripheral molecule, which is anchored to the outside of the membrane, or as an integral molecule that passes partway, or entirely, through the membrane. Based on what we discussed earlier with hydrophobicity and hydrophilicity, you may be able to guess that peripheral proteins have entirely hydrophilic outsides, while integral proteins contain at least one section that is hydrophobic and therefore hide from water with the tails. It's actually a little more complicated than that, but we'll discuss it in more detail later.

Next up is the nucleus, which is also enclosed in a plasma membrane very similar to the one surrounding the cell. The nucleus is responsible for containing the DNA. This is important because by walling off the DNA in its own compartment, the cell is better able to protect it from damage. Since our entire body is built off of the information encoded in DNA, damaged DNA leads to a variety of issues, the most notable of which is cancer. So as you can imagine, the nucleus serves a very important function. The membrane around the DNA is permeable to certain substances, such as hormones, which can act as messengers and tell the DNA to transcribe certain genes. This will be covered in more detail in the chapters on cell signaling and DNA replication.

Finally, the compartment between the nucleus and the cell membrane is the cytoplasm. All of the cell's organelles are found in the cytoplasm, and many reactions that take place in the cell occur in this environment. Because the cytoplasm is separated from the extracellular space by the plasma membrane, the environment inside the cell is different from the environment outside the cell. The cytoplasm is considered a reducing environment, which means that it can add electrons to molecules and make them more negative or less positive.

By contrast, the extracellular space is an oxidizing environment, which means that it takes away electrons and makes them more positive or less negative. This turns out to be important because molecules may take a different form within the cell than without, and they may also react differently inside the cell.

The organelles that can be found inside the cytoplasm include the endoplasmic reticulum, the Golgi apparatus, and mitochondria, among others. These organelles will be discussed in more detail in a later chapter.

Aside from the organelles, the cytoplasm contains two main components: the cytosol and the cytoskeleton. Now would probably be a good time to mention that in Greek, cyto- means cell, from the word *kutos,* meaning vessel or container. Most medical terms come from either Greek or Latin, so if you happen to speak either of those, you're way ahead of the game.

The cytosol is a fluid that bathes the organelles within the cytoplasm. This fluid is what allows the cell to be a reducing environment, as I mentioned earlier. While there is a lot of water within the cytosol, there are also hundreds of enzymes. Enzymes are molecules that help speed up a reaction without themselves being changed by a reaction. To understand this, think of making cookies in a bowl. If you tried to make cookies without a bowl, the process would be a lot more difficult and you'd probably lose a lot of ingredients to the floor, counter, etc. The bowl is an integral part of making the cookies, but it isn't really a part of the cookie-making and you still have a bowl at the end of the process. This isn't an exact analogy, since the enzymes do sometimes change form during a reaction and are converted back by the end of the reaction, but you get the idea.

These enzymes are used to metabolize most of the molecules that our body uses. Metabolism is the process by which we build up (anabolize) or break down (catabolize) molecules that are necessary for life. A good example of this is glucose, which we break down in our cells to produce energy (more on this when we talk about the mitochondria). In periods of fasting, we can also anabolize glucose in the liver to provide energy to the rest of our cells in a form they can use. As a general rule (though nothing in biology is 100%), catabolism takes place inside the mitochondria, while anabolism occurs in the cytoplasm.

That, in a nutshell, is the human cell. We'll now look at the major components in more detail.

DNA

Now that you understand the structure of the cell, it's time to look at each part in more detail. We'll start with the nucleus, since it contains the most important molecule in our entire body: DNA. DNA stands for deoxyribonucleic acid, and it is the basic building block of life. You can think of it as a blueprint for our bodies. DNA tells the manufacturing system of the cell what proteins to make, and these proteins are what handle a lot of the fun functions of our body. But what is DNA, exactly?

DNA is a double-stranded helix that resembles a ladder twisted from both ends like a rope. The sides of the ladder are made up of ribose sugars that have had an oxygen removed from one of the carbons, lending the "deoxyribo-" part of the name to DNA. These ribose sugars are pentamers that link together by way of a phosphate group. If these chemical names are getting to be too much, don't worry. This isn't actually the important part of DNA. The important part comes is the rungs that stretch across the ladder. Each rung is comprised of two bases, which are rings of carbons and nitrogens with oxygen attached. The two bases form hydrogen bonds, which is the same type of bond that water molecules form. These bonds are strong and hold the DNA together. There are four possible bases in DNA:

guanine, cytosine, adenine, and thymidine(which you'll also hear called thymine). One important thing about these bases is that each one can only connect with one other. Guanine and cytosine can link with each other, and adenine and thymidine can link with each other. No other combinations work, which turns out to be very important when it comes time to replicate the DNA. Because DNA is double-stranded, each strand of DNA has a complementary strand that contains the exact opposite bases. We'll talk about the significance of this when we get to the cell replication chapter.

Every single cell in our body has the same copy of DNA. In biology, there's something called the central dogma, which is this: DNA → RNA → protein. In other words, DNA gets transcribed into RNA, which gets translated into protein. RNA, or ribonucleic acid, is very similar to DNA in that it has a sugar backbone connected via phosphate groups, with bases coming off the side. The two main differences in humans are that instead of thymidine, one of the bases is uracil, and that RNA is single-stranded. This means that the strand can, and does, fold on itself to form bonds between the bases, but it doesn't have a complementary strand. The other difference is that RNA is only a very short segment compared to DNA. This occurs because DNA stores all of our genetic code, which as you can imagine, is way too much to be useful. It would be like trying to read through *War and Peace* each time you needed to find a single sentence in the book. Since DNA is far too long, memos get sent out in the form of RNA that encode for one protein. That protein is then assembled using the protein-making machine, also known as a ribosome (which also contains protein, confusingly).

To make DNA, we take those four bases mentioned earlier and combine them in various ways. Think of a set of blocks where you have countless blocks in only four colors: green, red, blue, and yellow. Although you only have four colors to choose from, you can combine them in any number of unique ways to make up unique segments of DNA called genes. For instance, you can take 5 red (R), 4 yellow (Y), 3 blue (B), and 1 green (G) to make: RRYGBRYYBRBRY, RYBRRRGYBYYRB, and countless other combinations. When you consider that you can change the number of each one of the four blocks, you start to realize that there are limitless ways you can arrange the DNA. Each of these combinations codes for a unique protein, so you can imagine that we can make a lot of proteins that do a lot of things in the body. There are about 3 billion base pairs in our genome, so the combinations are essentially limitless.

You've probably heard the terms "chromosome" and "genome" at various points throughout your life, and you're probably at least vaguely aware that they have something to do with DNA. A chromosome is a continuous, double-stranded piece of DNA. Rather than have one giant rope of DNA, the human body decided it would be more efficient to have 46 of them—23 from our mother, and 23 from our father. Each chromosome encodes hundreds of genes, which may or may not be related to each other. For instance, the gene that encodes for lactase—an enzyme that breaks down lactose so we can absorb it after we drink milk—is located on chromosome 2. There are also genes for collagen, desmin, and a lot of other proteins on chromosome 2. Chromosomes are numbered based on size, so that chromosome 1 is the largest and 22 is the smallest. You're probably wondering why I forgot chromosome 23, but the 23rd chromosome we get from our parents is the sex chromosome. These are only ever referred to as X and Y, so you won't hear about chromosome 23. This is because we have duplicates of the first 22, but half of the population has two distinct chromosomes for chromosome 23. Females all have two X chromosomes, but males have one X and one Y.

Since we get 23 of the chromosomes from our mother and 23 from our father, we actually have two of each gene. These genes aren't identical, however. The gene from our father often has a slightly different sequence than the one from your mother. Hair color is a good example of this: our parents often have slightly (or dramatically) different shades of hair color. The genes that code for hair still serve the same general function—producing hair—but small changes have given the hair different colors. The importance of duplicate genes is that we have a backup if something goes wrong. There are a lot of genetic disease that you'll hear referred to as "autosomal recessive" because they only occur when you get both copies of the mutated gene. "Autosomal" refers to chromosomes 1-22, which are the same in males and females. A good example of this is sickle cell anemia, in which the gene that codes for hemoglobin is affected. Hemoglobin is a protein found in red blood cells that carries oxygen to your tissues. Most people have the same sequence for this gene, but in a portion of the population, one nucleotide change means that they have a different amino acid in the sixth spot on the protein. We'll talk more about this when we get to the organelles chapter, but for now, all you need to understand is that you have a small change in the gene. If you only have one copy of this mutated gene, you don't typically have any symptoms of sickle cell disease and you may go through your entire life without ever knowing that you carry this mutation. This is, incidentally, why so many males are color-blind but females rarely are. That particular mutation is found on the X chromosome, and since females have two copies, even if one has the mutation, the other one works properly and makes up for the broken gene. Since males don't have a second X chromosome to compensate, they are color-blind. This is called "X-linked recessive" and refers to the fact that the mutation is on the X chromosome.

To understand the mutations, we need to delve a little further into the machinery of the cell. When discussing genetic codes, scientists abbreviate the bases to make writing the code simpler. So, for instance, if you had a gene that was made up of guanine, then adenine, then three cytosines, then two thymidines, it would be written like this: GACCCTT. The other convention that's used is that the code is always written in the 5' to 3' (pronounced 5 prime to 3 prime) direction. This leads me to the next point, which is, the directionality of DNA.

Deoxyribose is not a symmetrical molecule. The ring that makes up the body of deoxyribose contains one oxygen and four carbons, which are numbered 1-4 based on their proximity to the oxygen (not to mention the naming conventions of organic chemistry, which aren't worth getting into. The structure looks like this:

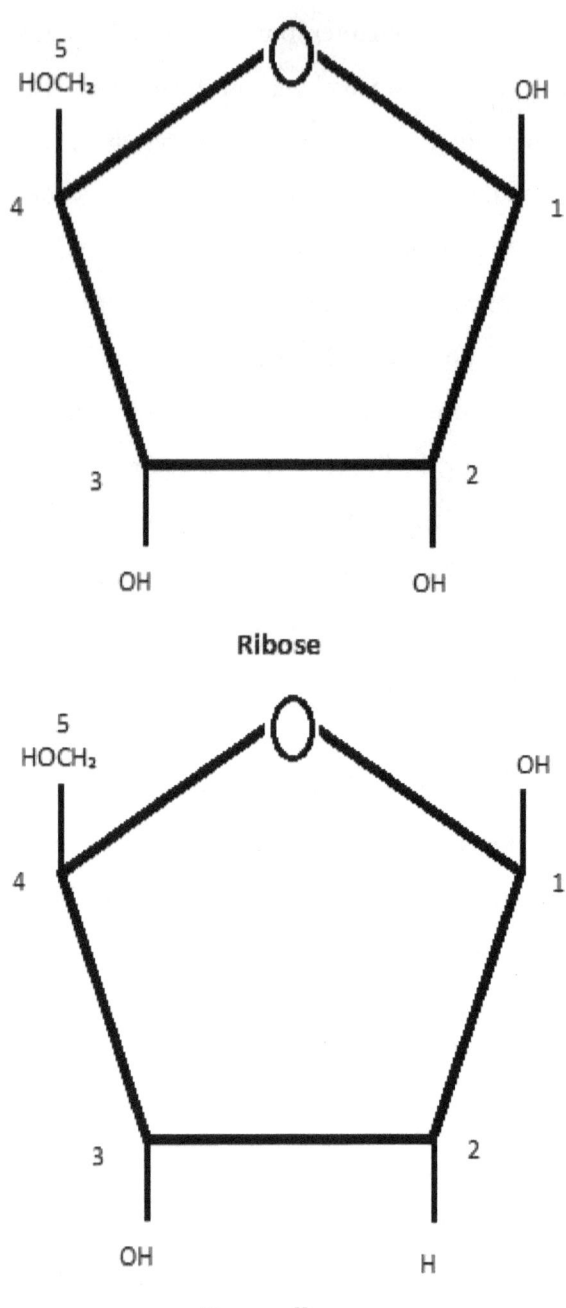

Ribose

Deoxyribose

If you look carefully, you can see that the 2' carbon on

deoxyribose is missing an oxygen. You also may notice that the 5' carbon isn't part of the ring, which is why it ends up getting labeled 5 instead of 1. This asymmetrical structure means that when the chain is formed, one 3' carbon links to a phosphate group, which links to a 5' carbon on a different deoxyribose ring. The chain is therefore directional, with one end having a free 5' carbon, and the other end having a free 3' carbon. The two strands that make up the double helix of DNA run in opposite directions, with the free 5' end of one strand paired with the free 3' end of the other.

So why do we care? We care because this turns out to be critical for DNA replication. Things get a little complicated here, so bear with me. It should all make sense at the end.

CELL REPLICATION

Overview

Cell replication occurs by a process called mitosis or meiosis. Mitosis is when a cell divides into two adult cells with all 46 chromosomes. Meiosis is the process by which we generate germ cells (sperm and eggs) that contain only half of our chromosomes (the other half come from the other parent). Replication occurs only when the environment is favorable, which the cell knows because of a series of complex signals that it receives from the extracellular environment. Once the cell decides to replicate, the chromosomes unwind and allow the DNA to be access so it can be copied in a process called replication. After the DNA is replicated, the chromosomes condense again and line up along a plane down the center of the cell. Identical copies of the same chromosome are held together in the center by a protein called a centromere. Fibers attached to each copy and pull the chromosomes to either side of the cell, dividing the DNA equally. The membrane that enclosed the nucleus then pinches shut in the middle, forming two separate nuclei. The cell then divides, with half of the cytoplasm and organelles going to each new cell. The two cells separate, and you're left with two identical cells.

If I haven't said this enough times, let me say it again: DNA is the blueprint of our bodies. This means it's the most important thing in our bodies, because if the blueprint gets altered, nothing will be produced properly. But in order to keep our bodies working, we need to have a mechanism for replacing cells that have been damaged. Now imagine someone hands you a book and a stack of blank paper and tells you to copy that book—five hundred times. On top of that, you can only write the second copy from the first copy, the third from the second, and so on. Maybe the first time through you'll be careful and make sure you don't miswrite something, but by the 436th time, there will probably be a lot of errors in your copies. This is basically what our body is doing, so you can see the challenge that our cells are up against. Luckily, our cell don't get bored or tired, and they have many mechanisms in place for ensuring proper replication.

Cells replicate through a carefully controlled process that responds to both intracellular and extracellular signals to decide if the replication is necessary and the environment is favorable. There are four phases to the cell cycle. The first, called Gap 1 (G1), occurs when the cell is resting, growing, and just generally doing whatever its function in the body is. There is an alternate phase during this time, called Gap 0 (G0), which is a phase that cells enter when they aren't replicating. Some cells become stuck in that phase forever, and these cells are said to be terminally differentiated. The muscle cells in our heart are a good example of these. Once our heart stops growing, the cells can never regenerate, even if some of them die because of loss of blood flow (and therefore oxygen) to those cells. This is exactly what happens in a heart attack (known as a myocardial infarction in medical speak), where blood flow stops to some of the cells, causing them to die. The cells that are left are stuck in G0 and therefore aren't able to replicate. Other cells, like the stem cells in our gut or skin, are able to leave G0 and get back into the cell replication cycle.

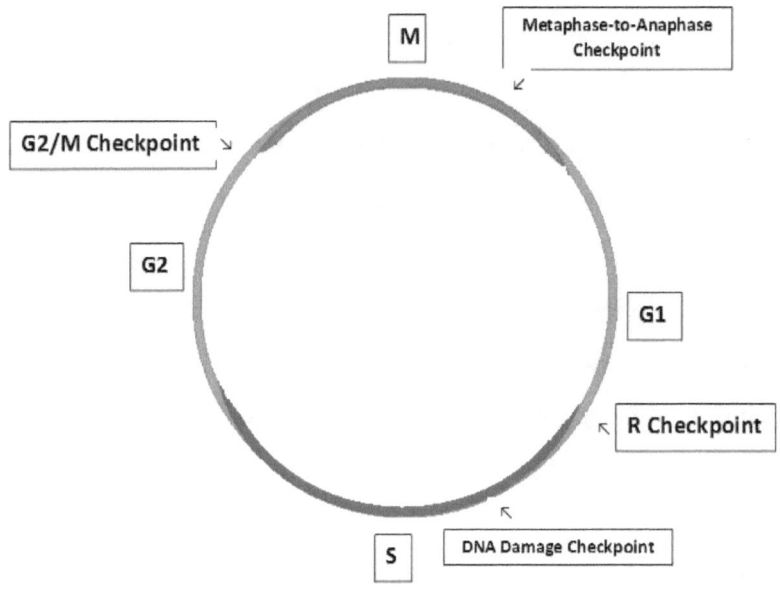

For our purposes right now, we're only going to focus on the cells that can get back into G1. G1 is essentially about getting ready to replicate and making sure that the cell has the resources to replicate. As the cell gets ready and reaches the end of G1, it hits a checkpoint called the restriction, or start, checkpoint. The progression past this checkpoint is controlled by molecules known as cyclins and cyclin-dependent kinases (CDKs). Understanding the expression of these molecules is well beyond the scope of this book, but what you should know is that extracellular signals cause cyclins and CDKs to be up- or down-regulated. The up-regulation of cyclin D and CDKs 4 and 6 allow the cell to progress past the R checkpoint into the S, or synthesis, phase (biochemists love to abbreviate everything).

The synthesis phase does exactly what you would expect—it synthesizes more DNA. In order to make another cell, you need to have two copies of DNA. Activation of cyclin A and cdk2 allows DNA synthesis to progress. This process, called replication, is done in a method known as semi-conservative; that is, the double-stranded DNA is separated into two different strands, and a second strand is synthesized onto each one. You end up with one strand of DNA from the old, parent DNA and one that is new, hence the name semi-conservative. But how is the strand copied?

As I mentioned earlier, the two DNA strands are exactly opposite to each other. Since each base can only pair with one other, we can know from looking at just one strand what the sequence of the opposite strand should be. Look at the following sequence, for example.

(5')AGGTTCTCACCT(3')
(3')TCCAAGAGTGGA(5')

If we see an adenine on one strand, we know that there must be a thymidine on the opposite strand. The same goes for guanine and cytosine. So even if we removed one strand, we could figure out the sequence by just knowing the one strand. Give it a try on this sequence (the correct answer is at the end of the chapter):

(5')TGCAGGTCACACATTG(3')

The thing that makes this slightly tricky is that you always see the sequence written 5' to 3', so if you had a grab-bag full of DNA sequences and had to pair up the correct complementary strands, the two strands from the first example would be written:

(5')AGGTTCTCACCT(3')   (5')AGGTGAGAACCT(3')

You might be wondering now why we always write the sequence from 5' to 3'. We do this because in human cells, DNA replication occurs 5' to 3'. No exceptions. This poses a challenge for the DNA replication machinery. The chromosomes in our cells are stored in a highly condensed form called chromatin. DNA is, amazingly, several meters long, so it has to be condensed in order to fit into the tiny nucleus of the cell. However, the condensed form is inaccessible to the DNA replication machinery. The first part of DNA replication is the decondensation of the chromatins.

Once this has occurred, a protein complex called the pre-replication complex (pre-RC) comes in and binds to a particular sequence of DNA called the origin of replication (ori). There are several thousand oris in human DNA, which is good because replicating that much DNA from only one ori would take a really, really long time. So during replication, multiple segments are being synthesized on the same strand. The pre-RC contains a protein called the minichromosome maintenance complex, which is thought to be responsible for holding the two old strands of DNA apart. Unless the parent strands are separated, no replication would be able to occur, so this is vital to replication success.

Think of DNA replication as pulling apart a zipper from the center of the zipper, rather than one end. This creates a so-called replication fork, where the two strands are separated to allow DNA synthesis to take place. The 5'-to-3' orientation becomes very important at this point because one strand runs from 5' to 3' toward the replication fork and can therefore be synthesized continuously, but the other one runs 3' to 5' and needs to be synthesized starting at the fork and moving away. This works fine for a short strand, but as the strand becomes more unzipped, there's a section of DNA that needs to be replicated but is on the wrong end of the DNA. Note that the template strand is read 3' to 5' in order to synthesize the complementary strand in a 5' to 3' direction.

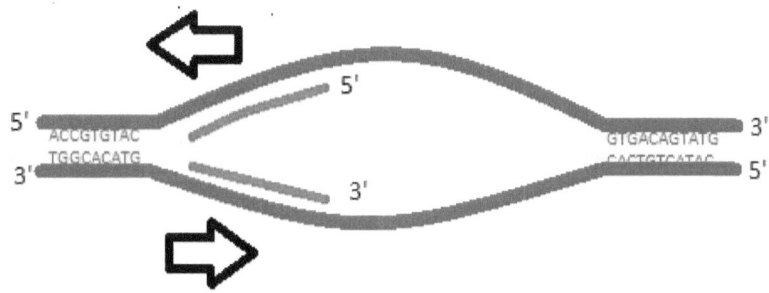

The strand at the bottom can progress and synthesize one big strand. This strand is called the leading strand We'll talk about that side first, then look at synthesis on the other strand, known as the lagging strand.

Once the pre-RC is attached, an enzyme known as primase comes in and synthesizes a short strand of complementary nucleotides that acts as a primer for the rest of the strand. This strand is composed of RNA rather than DNA, so it eventually needs to be replaced. At the same time, an enzyme known as DNA helicase comes to unwind the DNA ahead of the fork. As you may remember, DNA is stored in a twisted-ladder formation that doesn't lend itself to replication. Helicase breaks the bonds that are found between the matched pairs of nucleotides on either strand and separates the strands. Because DNA really prefers to be in a double-stranded formation, other proteins, known as single-stranded binding proteins (SSBs), bind to the separated nucleotides to prevent them from re-attaching to the other strand.

At this point, the replication of DNA is fairly straightforward. A protein known as DNA polymerase attaches to the leading strand and attaches the complement of the nucleotide on the leading strand to the strand being synthesized. If the leading strand has a guanine, then the DNA polymerase adds a cytosine to the new strand.

As replication proceeds, the strand gets more and more tightly wound ahead of the replication fork. This is fixed by DNA topoisomerase (yes, it's a protein) that cuts the strand all the way through, releasing some of the coils, and then seals it back together again.

Let's look at the lagging strand again. Since it needs to be synthesized in the 5' to 3' direction, the new strand is synthesized in a series of short fragments that are separated by a few bases (where the replication machinery was). These fragments are called Okazaki fragments and are named for the scientist who discovered their existence. The process is the same as the leading strand, but after replication is complete, the gaps need to be filled with nucleotides and sealed together. This is accomplished with the help of the replication complex, which removes the primers and replaces them with DNA. In case you're wondering, RNA is used at first because it can be synthesized without a primer, whereas DNA has to be added to an existing strand. Once you have all of the Okazaki fragments, the replication complex is able to add on to the fragments to replace the RNA primers. After that's complete, yet another protein, known as DNA ligase, comes in and seals the fragments together.

These multiple proteins work in sync to replicate DNA, making it a fairly smooth process. However, mistakes do occur—estimates range from 1,000 to 1,000,000 per cell per day. As you can imagine, if this many mistakes were left, our DNA would be completely different within a few months as we'd start to look like aliens. So DNA repair mechanisms are critical to our survival.

Before we get into the repair mechanisms, let's look at the types of mutations that occur. The first type is called a point mutation, and it happens when a single nucleotide is changed for another. For instance, the coding strand may have had a thymidine on it, but the DNA polymerase added a guanine to the strand instead of an adenine. These point mutations are further classified into silent, neutral, missense, and nonsense mutations, which we'll talk more about in the organelles chapter. The second and third mutation types are called insertion and deletion, and you can probably imagine what the mutation is—either an extra nucleotide (or nucleotides) is added, or one that should have been added is missed. Again, we'll talk about the implications in a bit, but these types of mutations can be extremely deleterious if they don't occur in sets of three. Finally, strand breaks can occur. These are usually caused by either UV exposure (like sunbathing for too long), exposure to certain chemicals, or viruses. The strand break can be either single-stranded, when only one half of the double helix breaks, or double-stranded, when the ladder completely snaps in half.

Now that I've convinced you mistakes do occur, let's discuss how our cells repair DNA. Since there are multiple types of mutations, there are multiple repair mechanisms as well: base excision repair (BER), nucleotide excision repair (NER), mismatch repair (MMR), homologous recombination (HR), and non-homologous end-joining (NHEJ).

We'll start by looking at mismatch repair because this is the primary mechanism for DNA errors that occur during replication. If the wrong base gets added to the growing strand of DNA during replication, DNA polymerase can look back one base and see if that the previous bases are incorrectly paired. If it attached an incorrect base—say, it added a thymidine instead of a cytosine—it backspaces, removing the incorrect nucleotide and attaching the correct one in its stead. This type of repair is very accurate because the system knows which strand is new and what base should have been added, so it can quickly add the right one.

Base excision repair occurs when a single base gets damaged. This can happen through exposure to free radicals or all sorts of other things that float around in our cells causing damage. Proteins called DNA glycosylases recognize the damaged base and chop it out of the strand, leaving the sugar-phosphate backbone in that spot. Another protein, called the AP endonuclease, cuts the bond on the backbone, and yet another protein removes the deoxyribose. Finally, a DNA polymerase comes in and adds a new, undamaged nucleotide.

Nucleotide excision repair is somewhat similar to base excision repair, but it's used when the damage is to multiple nucleotides. Typically this repair mechanism is used when damage is caused by UV light or chemicals that cause two or more nucleotides to link together. BER can't be used because that repair mechanism assumes that the damaged base can be cut away. If the base has fused with another base, cutting only the bonds that BER cuts won't free the nucleotide. NER is similar to DNA replication in that it unzips the double helix. It then chops away the damaged section, usually taking around thirty nucleotides out of that section just to make sure the damage is removed. The DNA polymerase then comes in and fills in the missing nucleotides using the undamaged strand as a template.

The final two mechanisms of repair are homologous recombination and non-homologous end-joining. HR is actually awesome in that it can work as both a repair mechanism and as a natural part of making eggs and sperm. It works by pairing up your two matching chromosomes—for instance, your two sets of chromosome 21—and either creating a double-stranded break or using one from DNA damage. The ends are then trimmed so that one strand is longer than the other. Since DNA bases really want to be in pairs, this makes the end "sticky", and so when another protein creates a gap between the strands on the other chromosome 21, the sticky end slides in and attempts to bond to that strand. Sometimes it works, sometimes it doesn't, and sometimes only a small piece of one chromosome 21 gets attached to the other chromosome 21. The cool thing about this is that if your body is repairing a broken strand, you know you have the same genes on your newly repaired strand. If it's being used to create eggs and sperm, the child can end up with a completely unique genome that neither parent has. Take, for instance, hair color. Hair color is coded for by multiple genes. For simplicity's sake, let's say that your mom has brown hair. She got a chromosome from her father that has two hair genes, one for brown hair and one that gives that hair a reddish tint. From her mom, she has a gene that would give her blond hair and another that gives that hair a reddish tint. When the two chromosomes cross over, the new chromosome created could end up with only the two genes for red hair. Depending on what genes you get from your father, you could end up with red hair, even if neither of your parents has red hair. And hair is just the beginning.

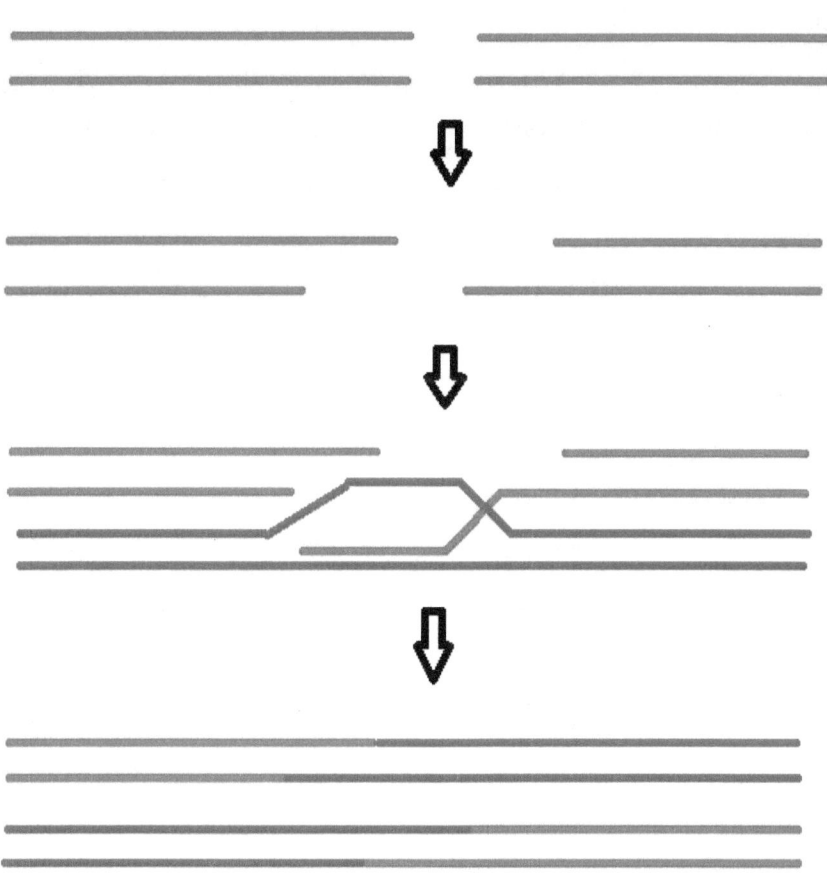

So that's homologous recombination. Non-homologous end-joining, on the other hand, is basically a last-ditch effort by your cells to fix themselves. The "homologous" part refers to the fact that the two chromosomes 21, in our previous example, encode for the same genes, though each chromosome you have may be slightly different in how those genes present. Non-homologous end-joining happens when a double-stranded break occurs in the chromosome and your body just grab another chromosome that also has a double-stranded break and fuses them together. The end result could be that three-quarters of chromosome 21 is still chromosome 21, but the last quarter is chromosome 5. This is better than not having an end to the chromosome and allows you to still express all of your genes, but sticking two random ends together could result in some very messed-up proteins.

And now, back to the cell cycle. As you can see, the S phase is a critical phase in cell replication because without DNA, the cell isn't much of a cell. After the S phase, the cell enters the Growth 2, or G2, phase. The G2 phase is fairly short and allows the cell a little time to grow, but its primary role is making sure the cell doesn't split in two until all of the DNA is replicated. The checkpoint at the end of G2, called the G2/M checkpoint or the DNA synthesis checkpoint, is regulated by yet more cyclins. In this case, cyclin B is bound to an inactive cdk1 until replication is complete. Once all the DNA synthesis is done, signals are sent that allow cdk1 to be activated, and the cell can then enter the mitosis, or M, phase.

Since biochemists love naming things, the M phase is further divided into four subphases of cell division, known as prophase, metaphase, anaphase, and telophase. Then some people got really clever and through in a prometaphase just because they felt like it. Here's how it works:

- **Prophase** – In this phase, the DNA begins to condense as much as possible. Identical copies of DNA, called sister chromatids, are held together by centromeres, making sure that they stay together as the DNA lines up for separation. Two proteins called centrosomes (since biochemists name everything, they run out of unique names after a while) move to either side of the nucleus so that they're 180 degrees from each other.

- **Prometaphase** – In this phase, the membrane surrounding the nucleus breaks down. Filaments known as kinetochores that are attached to centrosomes can now also attach to the chromosomes, and the chromosomes start to move around the cell to get lined up for division.
- **Metaphase** – The chromosomes line up along an equator halfway between the two centrosomes. Each sister chromatid attaches to a single kinetochore, and paired sister chromatids attach to kinetochores from opposite centrosomes.
- **Anaphase** – The kinetochores shorten, pulling the sister chromatids apart and moving them toward opposite sides of the cell.
- **Telophase** – The chromosomes reach opposite sides of the cell and new nuclear membranes form around the two sets of DNA, creating two separate nuclei in the cell. The cytoplasm of the cell starts to divide at this point as a contractile ring forms in the center of the cell and pinches inward.

When the contractile ring pinches all the way in, cytokinesis occurs, meaning that the cells completely separate. You're left with two cells containing identical DNA, ready to do their cellular duties.

Here's the answer to the DNA sequence problem from earlier

in the chapter:

(5')TGCAGGTCACACATTG(3')
(3')ACGTCCAGTGTGTAAC(5')

THE NUCLEUS

Cells do more than just replicate, and while the nucleus serves as a storage bin for DNA, a number of important cell processes take place inside the nucleus. The most important process that occurs here is DNA transcription. Transcription refers to the process by which DNA is copied to make RNA.

Before we get too far into the process of making RNA, it's important to know that there are a few different types of RNA. In the central dogma, in which DNA > RNA > protein, the RNA really refers to one type of RNA called messenger RNA (mRNA for short). The other significant types of RNA are transfer RNA (tRNA) and ribosomal RNA (rRNA). There are a few other types of RNA, but they're fairly insignificant and we don't entirely understand their functions, so we won't discuss them here.

The reason I say that we really mean mRNA when we say RNA is because mRNA contains the actual genetic sequence for the protein we're making. tRNA and rRNA are necessary to make the protein, but the protein code is contained within the mRNA. We'll delve into the functions of tRNA and rRNA when we discuss protein synthesis, but for now we're going to focus on the general process of synthesizing RNA.

RNA transcription occurs in a manner very similar to DNA replication, but only small portions of the DNA are transcribed into RNA. Just like DNA, RNA synthesis occurs in the 5' to 3' direction, with the template strand of DNA being read in the 3' to 5' direction. The main difference is that, since RNA is only a small piece of the DNA, there needs to be a way for the DNA to tell the transcription machinery where to start. This occurs through the use of a promoter sequence, which is a segment of DNA found 10-35 bases upstream from the DNA coding for the RNA to be transcribed. When RNA polymerase recognized this promoter region on the DNA, it binds there. The RNA polymerase is a complex of a number of proteins again just like DNA, that builds the RNA by adding one base at a time. Before the actual transcription can occur, though, a number of transcription factors are needed. Transcription factors interact with the DNA and either promote transcription, or inhibit it. This is one of the amazing things about our bodies because it allows our cells to control when certain proteins get made. As we discussed earlier, DNA gets transcribed to RNA, which is translated to proteins. If no mRNA is made, no proteins can be made from that RNA. RNA also has a limited lifespan, so even if we make lots of one type of RNA in response to some factor—for instance, if bacteria invade our body and the immune cells need to send out a lot of signals to recruit other immune cells—this will shut off after a pre-determined period of time. You can imagine how important this is, since some of the things our body does—like producing lots of immune cells and proteins to kill invaders—can actually be harmful to our own cells as well. If we couldn't turn off the production of proteins, we'd end up hurting ourselves.

Some RNA, known as constitutively expressed RNA, is made all the time, but a lot of RNA is transcribed in response to feedback mechanisms. This type is known as either inducible (meaning it can be turned on but isn't normally) or repressible (meaning it's normally made but can be shut off) RNA. For instance, the cyclins increase and decrease based on signals from the environment that tell the cell if it's ok to proceed or not. If the environment is unfavorable, the right signals aren't sent to the nucleus, the mRNA for cyclin D doesn't get transcribed, and the cell never progresses into the S phase. On the other hand, if the right signals are in place, cyclin D gets made, leading to further progression and more cyclin getting produced. Hopefully you can now see the beauty of this system, where we only produce proteins as we need them, allowing our cells to make different proteins in response to the body's needs. This is also how cells can specialize. Although the DNA in every cell is the same, certain cells only transcribe certain parts of the DNA. In our pancreas, we have cells known as beta cells that produce insulin. Other cells have the DNA for insulin, but it isn't active and never gets made into RNA, so those cells can't produce insulin.

After the right transcription factors are bound, the RNA polymerase moves down the DNA segment, adding ribose nucleotides, rather than deoxyribose, to the new strand of RNA. These ribose nucleotides contain almost the exact same bases as DNA and pair in the same manner, except RNA uses uracil (U) instead of thymidine.

The pairs are therefore C/G and A/U. When RNA polymerase reaches the end of the RNA segment, which it recognizes by mechanisms we still don't understand, a series of adenine nucleotides are added to the 3' end. This is known as a poly-A tail.

After the poly-A tail is added, you might think that the RNA segment is complete, but our body gets really tricky here. Instead of having the RNA perfectly match the DNA, only certain segments of the newly transcribed RNA will actually be used to make proteins. The RNA is composed of alternating segments known as introns and exons. Introns are parts of the RNA that get initially translated but are then cut out of the RNA molecule, leaving only the exons to be translated into proteins. This process occurs when a complex known as a spliceosome recognizes a GU sequence at the start of an intron and an AG at the end of the intron. It pulls the two segments together, cleaves the intron before the GU and after the AG, and sticks the two ends of the exons together. After this happens, a 5' "cap" is added, which helps stabilize the RNA and prevent degradation.

The interesting thing about this process is that in the end, only about 1.5% of our DNA actually codes for proteins. The rest is composed of introns and other non-coding regions. My theory on why this happens is that, as you recall, DNA mistakes happen all the time. If you have a lot of extraneous material, the mistakes may occur in that, rather than in the important bits. These mistakes might even turn non-coding regions into coding regions, producing a new protein that turns out to be useful for our survival. There are undoubtedly plenty of other reasons as well.

Since the nucleus is walled off from the rest of the cell, only certain molecules can actually pass into the nucleus. Since ribosomes are not one of them, the newly-transcribed RNA needs to be transported out of the nucleus. This occurs through nuclear pores, which are—you guessed it—proteins found in the nuclear membrane that allow substances to pass through. The destination of the RNA is either to the cytoplasm or the endoplasmic reticulum, one of the organelles found in the cell that we'll be discussing next.

ORGANELLES

Endoplasmic Reticulum

The endoplasmic reticulum (ER) is essentially a network of membranes folded in on itself that surrounds the nucleus and is continuous with the membrane of the nucleus. It resembles a hedge maze, with a series of folded sacs called cisternae that provide a membrane surface for a number of critical cell activities. The cisternae hold proteins that are waiting to be modified and sent to the appropriate places.

There are two types of ER: rough ER and smooth ER. The rough ER is so named because its membranous surface is studded with ribosomes. You may recall from earlier that ribosomes are the protein-making machinery of a cell. The rough ER, therefore, is where protein synthesis takes place. This makes sense, given the function of the cisternae for modifying and storing proteins. It's far easier for the cell to make protein right next to where it's modified than to ship it across the cell.

The smooth ER, on the other hand, serves as a detoxification site in many cells, as well as a site of sequestration for calcium ions. In cells that secrete steroids, the smooth ER is the site of steroid and lipid synthesis. When I say steroids, I don't mean anabolic steroids that bodybuilders take; steroids are a hormone produced in our bodies. The SER is important in the liver, which is a major site of detoxification in our bodies. For the purposes of this book, this is the extent of what you need to know about the smooth ER.

The amount of ER that can be found in any given cell is largely dependent on the function of the cell. Cells in the human body specialize to perform a wide variety of functions. Cells that primarily make protein, for instance, contain a large amounts of rough ER. A good example of this is cells found in the pancreas that are responsible for making the enzymes we use to digest food. Since enzymes are proteins, these cells have a large amount of rough ER when compared to other cells.

We'll look at the rough ER and protein synthesis first. Protein synthesis can also occur in the cytoplasm. The function of the protein determines where it is synthesized. Proteins that will stay in the cytoplasm, such as enzymes that are used in making fatty acids, are synthesized in the cytoplasm. Proteins that will span a membrane, such as the nuclear pores we discussed earlier, are made in the rough ER. This is done not only for efficiency, but also because those transmembrane proteins generally have a hydrophobic section that doesn't want to be near the cytoplasm, and the hydrophobic tails of the lipids in the membrane of the rough ER provide a safe haven for those proteins.

So how is protein made? As we discussed earlier, protein is made from RNA, and specifically from mRNA. Once mRNA is made, it's sent out of the nucleus to the rough ER. Protein synthesis starts when the ribosome complex binds to the mRNA molecule. Ribosome complexes are composed of two protein subunits, termed 60S and 40S, and 4 rRNA molecules. The 40S subunit and one rRNA strand recognize the start codon on the mRNA molecule, which is always the sequence AUG (remember that uracil has replaced thymidine on RNA).

Before we go further, there are a few things you need to know. The first is that RNA is translated into proteins by creating a chain of amino acids, called a peptide chain. Multiple peptide chains can then be folded into a single protein. Amino acids are molecules composed of carbon, oxygen, nitrogen, hydrogen, and a variable group. There are twenty amino acids that are used to make proteins in humans; there are other amino acids as well, but only twenty of them are used to make proteins. These amino acids can be neutral, basic, acidic, hydrophobic, and small or large. We can synthesize eleven of these in our bodies, but nine of them are termed "essential" amino acids because we have to get them from our diets. These essential amino acids are what people mean when they say you need to get protein in your diet, because when we eat protein, our body breaks down the peptide chains that make up the protein into amino acids. The main source is, of course, meat, but you can also get these amino acids from eggs, beans, rice, and a variety of other sources.

The second thing to know is that the ribosomes know what amino acid to add to the chain based on a three-nucleotide sequence known as a codon. AUG always starts the chain, and that tells the ribosome what frame to read. Remember when I mentioned that insertions and deletions were really bad if they didn't occur in sets of three? This is why. If you delete one nucleotide, the ribosome will read the first nucleotide in the next codon as the third nucleotide in the codon that has the missing nucleotide. Everything after that spot will be shifted over one, making the rest of the mRNA into a giant strand of gibberish.

The third thing to know is that each codon only codes for one amino acid, but there are multiple codons for each amino acid.

Amino Acid	Codons	Properties
Glycine	GGU, GGC, GGA, GGG	Small
Alanine	GCU, GCC, GCA, GCG	Small
Serine	UCU, UCC, UCA, UCG, AGU, AGC	Polar uncharged
Threonine	ACU, ACC, ACA, ACG	Polar uncharged
Cysteine	UGU, UGC	Sulfur
Valine	GUU, GUC, GUA, GUG	Hydrophobic
Leucine	UUA, UUG, CUU, CUC, CUA, CUG	Hydrophobic
Isoleucine	AUU, AUC, AUA	Hydrophobic
Methionine	AUG (always starts chain)	Hydrophobic
Proline	CCU, CCC, CCA, CCG	Hydrophobic
Phenylalanine	UUU, UUC	Hydrophobic
Tyrosine	UAU, UAC	Hydrophobic
Tryptophan	UGG	Hydrophobic
Aspartic Acid	GAU, GAC	Negatively charged
Glutamic Acid	GAA, GAG	Negatively charged
Asparagine	AAU, AAC	Polar uncharged
Glutamine	CAA, CAG	Polar uncharged
Histidine	CAU, CAC	Positively charged
Lysine	AAA, AAG	Positively charged
Arginine	CGU, CGC, CGA, CGG, AGA, AGG	Positively charged

This means that GGU will always code for glycine, but GGC, GGA, and GGG can also be used to get the same amino acid. You may notice that the start codon AUG also codes for methionine, so it always starts the peptide chain. Proteins are typically processed before they get sent anywhere, so they don't all always have methionine at the beginning. If you're really sharp, you may have noticed that there's a start codon but not a stop codon. There are, in fact, three stop codons: UAA, UAG, and UGA; they just don't code for any amino acids.

Think back to our discussion of point mutations during DNA synthesis. We can now understand the different types of mutations and how they affect the protein. Take the codon UAU, for example. If the second uracil in this sequence were accidentally switched to a cytosine (UAC), the codon would still code for tyrosine. This is called a silent mutation because it doesn't cause any sort of change in the protein. If the adenine were switched out for a uracil (UUU), though, this would change the amino acid to phenylalanine. Because phenylalanine is hydrophobic, just like tyrosine, the effect it has on the protein would be negligible. When a mutation causes an amino acid to be exchanged for another, similar amino acid, we call that a neutral mutation. Aspartic acid changing to glutamic acid would be another example. Let's say our first nucleotide gets changed, though, going from a uracil to a guanine (GAU). This would cause an aspartic acid, which is negatively charged, to be added to the protein in place of the tyrosine. Since tyrosine is hydrophobic and aspartic acid is hydrophilic, this could change the way the protein functions. Say the tyrosine was in the middle of a series of amino acids that were all hydrophobic and were intended to be inside the membrane. Having a hydrophilic amino acid in there would be problematic because it wants to be outside the membrane, not hiding inside it. This is called a missense mutation, and it's the type of mutation that occurs in sickle cell anemia. So you can see how even one change can be deleterious to our health.

The final type of mutation is called a nonsense mutation. This happens when a codon is accidentally changed to a stop codon. If the last letter of our UAU sequence were changed to an A or a G, we would have a stop codon. Now imagine this codon is the sixth codon in an mRNA molecule that codes for a 250-amino-acid-long protein. We would stop translating almost as soon as we started, and there's no way for the ribosomes to start up again. In that case, we completely lack whatever protein was being coded for, and we have to hope it wasn't an important one.

Now that we understand amino acids and mutations a little better, let's get back to the protein synthesis. So far we have a 40S subunit and one rRNA binding to the AUG on the mRNA. The 40S subunit has two other sites of import—a "P" site, so named for the fact that it holds the growing peptide chain; and an "A" site, named because the amino acids bind at this site. After the 40S subunit attaches to the mRNA, a tRNA comes in, attached to an amino acid.

You might be wondering how and why the tRNA got a hold of an amino acid. tRNA molecules are short segments (typically 74-95 nucleotides in length), shaped like a 3-leaf clover, that contain a few conserved regions and one variable one. The conserved regions are one arm that can bind to the ribosome, known as the ribothymidine pseudouridine cytidine arm (I did not make this up. This is what biochemists like to do to us), and an arm that can bind to one specific amino acid, known more appropriately as the acceptor arm. The variable region is known as the anticodon region, and it contains three nucleotides that are the complement to the codon for the amino acid it holds. A tRNA that can bind to tryptophan, for example, would have ACC as its anticodon—the exact opposite of UGG. Each tRNA molecule can only bind to one type of amino acid, and our body naturally has a mechanism in place for ensuring the tRNA binds to the right amino acid.

For the first amino acid, the tRNA comes in and binds to the P site of the ribosome. The tRNA can only bind if its anticodon complements the codon in the P site. This is the manner by which the mRNA is "read" and the protein is synthesized correctly. The only exception is that there's a little wiggle room on the last letter, so as long as the first two match, a tRNA can usually bind. This is generally ok because most of the codons that have the same two first letters are for the same, or a similar, amino acid.

Once the first tRNA is bound, the 60S subunit with its three rRNA molecules comes in and helps stabilize the entire ribosome. After the complex is stabilized, another tRNA—with the appropriate anticodon—binds to the A site. A bond forms between the two amino acids, and the entire ribosome complex slides down one spot. The A site becomes the P site and the P-site tRNA is released. A new A site opens up and another tRNA comes in, and the process repeats itself. This goes on until the end of the mRNA is reached. At that point, the protein can fold on itself, get processed further, or join with a few other peptide chains to form a complete protein.

Golgi Apparatus and Secretory Granules

If the Golgi apparatus were a villain in a sci-fi movie, it would be The Blob. The Golgi apparatus is composed of a series of membranous saccules whose primary function is to secrete transport vesicles that materials being shipped elsewhere in the cell. The Golgi has two sides, a *cis* face and a *trans* face. The *cis* face is near the rough ER and receives materials (often proteins) that need to be packaged and sent somewhere else. The Golgi is also a site of protein modification, which occurs as the proteins pass through to the *trans* side. At the *trans* face, a number of mechanisms regulate the assembly of proteins into secretory granules.

Secretory granules, as you might imagine, are vesicles that store some product, waiting for a signal to release it. A good example of this is in neuronal junctions, which store neurotransmitters in vesicles, waiting for the cell to depolarize. When the cell depolarizes, the vesicles fuse with the cell membrane and dump their contents into the gap between neurons. While secretory granules assemble in the Golgi apparatus, they can wait anywhere in the cell, typically near the membrane. The beauty of this system is that you can pre-make the substance you need and be able to release it instantaneously. That way, when you need that neurotransmitter, you don't have to wait for your DNA to be transcribed to RNA and then translated into the proteins you need.

Mitochondria

In my opinion, mitochondria (singular mitochondrion) are the coolest thing in our entire bodies. They're unique in that unlike any other organelle, they contain their own DNA. The prevailing theory on why they have their own DNA is that over a billion years ago, mitochondria were bacteria that were engulfed by eukaryotic cells. The mitochondria were able to provide cellular energy by the mechanism we'll discuss in a minute, and the eukaryotic cell provided them a safe, warm environment in which to live.

The other cool thing about mitochondrial DNA is that it only comes from your mother. The reason for this is that sperm need to be small in order to be motile, so they only contain DNA and drop most of the unnecessary organelles. The egg, on the other hand, is much larger and doesn't have to move, so it contains mitochondria. This is true no matter how far back you go—your mother's mother had the same mitochondrial DNA, and her mother, and so on back to the beginning of time. A prominent geneticist actually wrote a book about mitochondrial DNA called *The Seven Daughters of Eve*, a book I found at a hostel in Scotland and then spent most of my vacation there reading it instead of exploring Scotland.

Mitochondria are Mike-and-Ike-shaped structures that contain an inner, folded membrane surrounded by the outer membrane. The space between the inner and outer membranes is called the intermembrane space. The folds of the inner membrane are known as cristae, and the space inside the inner membrane is the central matrix.

The primary role of mitochondria is to serve as the so-called "energy factory" of the cell. They do this by producing adenosine triphosphate (ATP), which contains high-energy bonds that can be broken to provide energy for reactions to occur. Remember earlier when we talked about anabolism and catabolism, and I mentioned that most catabolism takes place inside the mitochondria? This is so we can harness the energy for the molecules being broken down in order to produce ATP.

I'm sure you're familiar with the basic concept that we get our energy from food. You also know that we don't eat constantly, so we must have a way of storing energy to use when we aren't eating. We have a number of mechanisms for this, actually, including fat storage, but for short-term storage, we turn to ATP. Let's look at that glucose molecule from earlier. Once it moves out of our gut and into our cells, it gets sent to the mitochondria. There, it's broken into two pyruvate molecules, which enter something known as the citric acid cycle, Krebs cycle, or the TCA cycle (short for tricarboxylic acid cycle). Through this cycle, we produce a net 2 ATP and release a few electrons, which can then be sent through something called the electron transport chain. The energy from those electrons gains us an addition 32 ATP. However, the electron transport chain can only run in the presence of oxygen, so during periods of heavy exercise when we don't have enough oxygen going to our muscles, those electrons are used to produce only a few more ATP and release lactic acid. If you've ever worked out and had sore muscles afterward, you're familiar with lactic acid.

Mitochondria also take part in cell death, which you'll see soon.

Lysosomes

Lysosomes are small, membrane-bound vesicles that serve as sites of intracellular digestion. The enzymes they contain vary depending on what substances they break down, and they're found in large quantities in cells like macrophages, which are the scavengers of our body that ingest and destroy bacteria before it can infect us. Lysosomal enzymes can break down almost anything that we throw at them, much like a garbage disposal. Because lysosomes are pretty indiscriminate about what they break down, our cells did two ingenious things to make sure the lysosomes don't start digesting us. First, the lysosomes are surrounded by a membrane, segregating the enzymes from the rest of the cell. Second, most of the enzymes work at a pH lower (more acidic) than the pH found in our cells—they work around 5.0, but the cytosol typically has a pH around 7.2. If lysosomal enzymes leak out, they become inactivated in the more basic environment and can't do any damage.

Like secretory granules, lysosomal enzymes are packaged in the Golgi apparatus and shipped out into the cytosol. There, lysosomes wait for material to be sent its way. If the debris comes from outside the cell, the cell engulfs in and pinches off a portion of the cellular membrane to form a phagosome (Greek *phago:* to eat). This process is called endocytosis. The phagosome then fuses with the lysosome to form one big, happy phagolysosome. The enzymes inside the phagolysosome break down the debris, and the nutrients that are released actually diffuse across the lysosomal membrane to be used by the cell for energy. Isn't our body clever?

Sometimes indigestible material remains, and this is called a residual body. Residual bodies can actually be seen on slides under a microscope and can indicate cell damage.

Lysosomes can also digest unwanted parts of the cell, such as damaged or excess organelles, through a process called autophagy. The smooth ER forms a membrane around the item to be digested and fuses with the lysosome. From there, the process is the same as in the phagolysosome. In times of starvation, the cell will actually begin to eat itself in order to get energy.

Proteasomes

Proteasomes are small proteins that function to break down other proteins. They are not enclosed in a membrane and can therefore work freely in the cell. However, proteasomes don't degrade proteins willy-nilly. Instead, they can only recognize proteins with a particular molecule, called ubiquitin, attached. Ubiquitin molecules are attached to misfolded proteins by yet more proteins, essentially adding a handle for proteasomes to grab onto. The proteasome then breaks down the peptide into short chains that can be reused for protein synthesis or sent elsewhere as needed.

Peroxisomes

Peroxisomes are, once again, membrane-enclosed organelles. They're named because of their enzymes, which make, and then break down, hydrogen peroxide. You're probably wondering why our cells would do that. The process of producing hydrogen peroxide is part of a process of inactivating toxic molecules, including prescription drugs. The enzymes, called oxidases, add an oxygen molecule to water, producing hydrogen peroxide (H_2O_2). Because hydrogen peroxide is toxic to cells, the peroxisomal enzymes immediately break it down. This may sound silly, but deficiencies in peroxisomes can actually lead to medical problems such as Zellweger Syndrome, which affects many organ systems, including the brain.

CELL SIGNALING

With billions of cells in our body working in tandem to keep us alive, our cells need multiple methods for communicating in order to keep things running smoothly. We'll look at the basics of this communication.

Cells that are adjacent to one another can communicate through gap junctions, which are protein channels found in the membranes of cells. The protein passes through the membranes of both cells, creating an opening that allows small molecules and ions such as sodium and calcium to pass through, while keeping the larger molecules contained to their respective cells. The heart is a good example of cells that communicate through gap junctions. When one cell contracts, calcium flows through the gap junctions and causes all of the cells to contract simultaneously, which is critical in order to pump blood throughout our body. This is an efficient way for nearby cells to communicate because the communication is essentially instantaneous, but you can probably imagine that it isn't a particularly effective method for cells that are further apart.

So how do the cells in your finger communicate with the cells in your feet? These types of signals occur through the use of signal molecules that bind with receptor proteins on the surface of the cell.

You may recall that the membrane is studded with proteins, many of which cross through the membrane and have portions on both the intracellular and extracellular sides. Some of these proteins are receptors. There are thousands of types of receptors in our bodies, and the exact conformation of the protein determines what signal molecule can bind to it. Cells that contain a receptor for a particular signal molecule are called target cells. A good example of this is thyroid-stimulating hormone (TSH), which binds to thyrotropin receptors on the thyroid cells and signals for them to produce more thyroid hormone. Since other cells don't have the TSH receptor, only thyroid cells can respond to this particular stimulus.

Signals are divided into a number of categories based on the route they take to get to the target cell. These categories are autocrine, paracrine, synaptic, endocrine, and juxtacrine signaling. Autocrine signaling takes place when a cell releases a signal molecule that then binds to a receptor on that same cell. Paracrine signaling occurs when the signal molecules bind to receptors on nearby cells. Endocrine signals, on the other hand, travel through the blood to reach target cells that may be anywhere in the body. Synaptic is a type of paracrine signaling but only occurs in the synapses of nerves. Finally, juxtacrine signaling occurs when a signal molecule on a cell membrane binds to a receptor protein on the target cell.

When the signal molecule binds to the receptor protein, a series of events occurs inside the cell that tells the cell how to react. Some signal molecules bind to ion channels and open or close the channels, allowing ions to flow into (or stop flowing into/out of) a cell. This is the type of signal seen in neurons. Other types, such as G-protein coupled and receptor tyrosine kinases, are attached to molecules inside the cell. When the signal molecule binds to the receptor, it causes the receptor protein to change shape. This shape change leads to a change in the molecule attached to the receptor, setting off a chain of events known as the second messenger cascade. The second messengers are released and move to their target within the cell. Different molecules are bound to different receptors and therefore have different targets based on the receptor that was activated.

As I'm sure you can imagine, things go horribly wrong when cells don't respond properly to outside signals. One example is dwarfism, where the growth hormone receptor is dysfunctional. Without the receptor, the cells can't respond properly to growth hormone and the person therefore doesn't grow.

CELL DEATH

As with all things, our cells, too, must die. This was a concept that puzzled me when I first started to learn about the cell because some cells, such as those in the gut, only have a lifespan of 4-6 days. I didn't understand how humans could live for decades when our cells couldn't even last a week. You may recall me mentioning stem cells earlier. These are the cells from which our bodies regenerate old cells. Stem cells are protected from the exposure to potentially toxic factors, so they're much less likely to be damaged than the cells at the surface of our small intestine, which are constantly exposed to the chemicals and bacteria we ingest. Cells such as these can therefore survive our entire lifetime and provide a pool from which to replenish our more frequently damaged cells through mitosis. The cells that are getting damaged, on the other hand, die off quickly. But how do they die?

There are two types of cell death: apoptosis and necrosis. Of the two, apoptosis is infinitely preferred because it occurs in a nice, clean manner that doesn't cause problems. Apoptosis is often known as programmed cell death because it follows a pre-programmed pattern for eliminating bad cells. Necrosis, on the other hand, means something went wrong. This is what happens in a heart attack or stroke where oxygen supply to the cells is lost. Instead of undergoing a nice, clean death, the cells burst and spill their contents everywhere, causing more damage to the cells around them. We'll look at each one in more detail.

Apoptosis occurs in two instances. The first is when we're growing fetuses in the womb. Fetuses overproduce certain cells at different periods that are necessary for only a short while. Once that time is past, the cells die through apoptosis. In adults, apoptosis only occurs when DNA suffers irreparable damage. You probably recall from the chapter on cell division that our bodies have numerous repair mechanisms for DNA damage. When all of these fail, certain signals get activated, telling the cell to die.

Signals for apoptosis can occur via an extracellular pathway and an intracellular pathway. In the extracellular pathway, a signal molecule called Fas binds to the Fas receptor on the surface of the cell. This activates the Fas-associated death domain (FADD), which in turn activates caspases. More on caspases in a minute.

The intracellular pathway occurs when mitochondria release a molecule known as cytochrome c. Mitochondria release cytochrome c in response to signals sent telling the mitochondria that the DNA is damaged. Once cytochrome c is released, it binds to apoptosis activating factor 1 (Apaf-1), and the two activate caspases.

As you can see, caspases are the point where both pathways converge. The role of caspases is to chop up DNA into little bits. They also assist in condensation of the cytoplasm and chromatin. The final step in apoptosis is membrane blebbing, where the cell breaks apart into small globules that can then be eaten by other cells and digested in their lysosomes for nutrients. Throughout the process, the contents of the cell are contained and can't cause damage to neighboring cells.

The downfall of apoptosis from a cellular perspective is that it requires energy to proceed. If energy runs out, such as when oxygen supply is cut off and the mitochondria can't produce all that ATP, necrosis occurs. Unfortunately, we still aren't entirely sure of the mechanism of necrosis. What is known, though, is that the cells break down and spill their contents into the extracellular space, rather than blebbing off into small packages that can be cleanly digested by other cells. This can cause damage to the neighboring cells, such as when enzymes that break down proteins are released and can access the proteins in the other cell membranes. When necrosis occurs, the death can spread to neighboring cells through the damage they cause. Overall, this is a mechanism we try to avoid.

CONCLUSION

As you now can see, the cell is an incredibly complex system inside of an even more complex system: the human body. In this book, we've touched on the basics of cell function, replication, and death, but it's fair to say that we've only brushed the surface. Many researchers dedicate their entire lives to researching just one small part of the cell. The discoveries they've made have allowed us to produce medicines that can change the course of a disease or destroy invading bacteria without hurting our cells. In future years, we may see great progress in treating cancer, heart disease, and a plethora of other diseases as we come to understand the pathways that take place inside the human body.

SOURCES

Barrett KE, Boitano S, Barman SM, Brooks HL. Chapter 2. Overview of Cellular Physiology in Medical Physiology. In: Barrett KE, Boitano S, Barman SM, Brooks HL. eds. GANONG'S REVIEW OF MEDICAL PHYSIOLOGY, 24E. New York, NY: McGraw-Hill;
2012. http://accessmedicine.mhmedical.com.ezproxy.fau.edu/content.aspx?bookid=393&Sectionid=39736740. Accessed May 17, 2015.

Brooks GF, Carroll KC, Butel JS, Morse SA, Mietzner TA. Chapter 2. Cell Structure. In: Brooks GF, Carroll KC, Butel JS, Morse SA, Mietzner TA. eds.JAWETZ, MELNICK, & ADELBERG'S MEDICAL MICROBIOLOGY, 26E. New York, NY: McGraw-Hill;
2013.http://accessmedicine.mhmedical.com.ezproxy.fau.edu/content.aspx?bookid=504&Sectionid=40999921. Accessed January 09, 2015.

Haldar SM, Walsh RA. Chapter 7. Molecular and Cellular Biology of the Normal, Hypertrophied, and Failing Heart. In: Fuster V, Walsh RA, Harrington RA. eds.HURST'S THE HEART, 13E. New York, NY: McGraw-Hill;
2011.http://accessmedicine.mhmedical.com.ezproxy.fau.edu/content.aspx?bookid=376&Sectionid=40279732. Accessed May 19, 2015.

Jameson J, Kopp P. Chapter 61. Principles of Human Genetics. In: Longo DL, Fauci AS, Kasper DL, Hauser SL, Jameson J, Loscalzo J. eds. HARRISON'S PRINCIPLES OF INTERNAL MEDICINE, 18E. New York, NY: McGraw-Hill;
2012.http://accessmedicine.mhmedical.com.ezproxy.fau.edu/content.aspx?bookid=331&Sectionid=40726790. Accessed May 11, 2015.

Janson LW, Tischler ME. Chapter 9. DNA/RNA Function and Protein Synthesis.In: Janson LW, Tischler ME. eds. THE BIG PICTURE: MEDICAL BIOCHEMISTRY. New York, NY: McGraw-Hill;
2012.http://accessmedicine.mhmedical.com.ezproxy.fau.edu/content.aspx?bookid=397&Sectionid=39898615. Accessed May 11, 2015.

Kemp WL, Burns DK, Brown TG. Chapter 1. Cellular Pathology. In: Kemp WL, Burns DK, Brown TG. eds. PATHOLOGY: THE BIG PICTURE. New York, NY: McGraw-Hill;
2008. http://accessmedicine.mhmedical.com.ezproxy.fau.edu/content.aspx?bookid=499&Sectionid=41568284. Accessed May 19, 2015.

Mescher AL. Chapter 2. The Cytoplasm. In: Mescher AL. eds. JUNQUEIRA'S BASIC HISTOLOGY: TEXT & ATLAS, 13E. New York, NY: McGraw-Hill; 2013.http://accessmedicine.mhmedical.com.ezproxy.fau.edu/content.aspx?bookid=574&Sectionid=42524588. Accessed April 29, 2015.

Mescher AL. Chapter 5. Connective Tissue. In: Mescher AL. eds. JUNQUEIRA'S BASIC HISTOLOGY: TEXT & ATLAS, 13E. New York, NY: McGraw-Hill; 2013.http://accessmedicine.mhmedical.com.ezproxy.fau.edu/content.aspx?bookid=574&Sectionid=42524591. Accessed April 19, 2015.

Mescher AL. Chapter 9. Nerve Tissue & the Nervous System. In: Mescher AL.eds. JUNQUEIRA'S BASIC HISTOLOGY: TEXT & ATLAS, 13E. New York, NY: McGraw-Hill;
2013. http://accessmedicine.mhmedical.com.ezproxy.fau.edu/content.aspx?bookid=574&Sectionid=42524595. Accessed April 19, 2015.

Murray RK, Weil P. Membranes: Structure & Function. In: Rodwell VW, Bender DA, Botham KM, Kennelly PJ, Weil P. eds. HARPER'S ILLUSTRATED BIOCHEMISTRY, 30E. New York, NY: McGraw-Hill; 2015.http://accessmedicine.mhmedical.com.ezproxy.fau.edu/content.aspx?bookid=1366&Sectionid=73245687. Accessed April 19, 2015.

Paulsen DF. Chapter 2. The Plasma Membrane & Cytoplasm. In: Paulsen DF.eds. HISTOLOGY & CELL BIOLOGY: EXAMINATION & BOARD REVIEW, 5E. New York, NY: McGraw-Hill; 2010.http://accessmedicine.mhmedical.com.ezproxy.fau.edu/content.aspx?bookid=563&Sectionid=42045295. Accessed January 04, 2015.

Paulsen DF. Chapter 4. Epithelial Tissue. In: Paulsen DF. eds. HISTOLOGY & CELL BIOLOGY: EXAMINATION & BOARD REVIEW, 5E. New York, NY: McGraw-Hill; 2010.http://accessmedicine.mhmedical.com.ezproxy.fau.edu/content.aspx?bookid=563&Sectionid=42045298. Accessed April 19, 2015.

Paulsen DF. Chapter 10. Muscle Tissue. In: Paulsen DF. eds. HISTOLOGY & CELL BIOLOGY: EXAMINATION & BOARD REVIEW, 5E. New York, NY: McGraw-Hill; 2010.http://accessmedicine.mhmedical.com.ezproxy.fau.edu/content.aspx?bookid=563&Sectionid=42045304. Accessed April 19, 2015.

Weil P. Chapter 36. RNA Synthesis, Processing, & Modification. In: Murray RK, Bender DA, Botham KM, Kennelly PJ, Rodwell VW, Weil P. eds. HARPER'S ILLUSTRATED BIOCHEMISTRY, 29E. New York, NY: McGraw-Hill; 2012.http://accessmedicine.mhmedical.com.ezproxy.fau.edu/content.aspx?bookid=389&Sectionid=40142514. Accessed May 09, 2015.

Weil P. Protein Synthesis & the Genetic Code. In: Rodwell VW, Bender DA, Botham KM, Kennelly PJ, Weil P. eds. HARPER'S ILLUSTRATED BIOCHEMISTRY, 30E.New York, NY: McGraw-Hill; 2015.http://accessmedicine.mhmedical.com/content.aspx?bookid=1366&Sectionid=73245262. Accessed May 08, 2015.

www.ingramcontent.com/pod-product-compliance
Lightning Source LLC
Chambersburg PA
CBHW021025180526
45163CB00005B/2121